DELICIOUS ANTI-CANCER SMOOTHIES

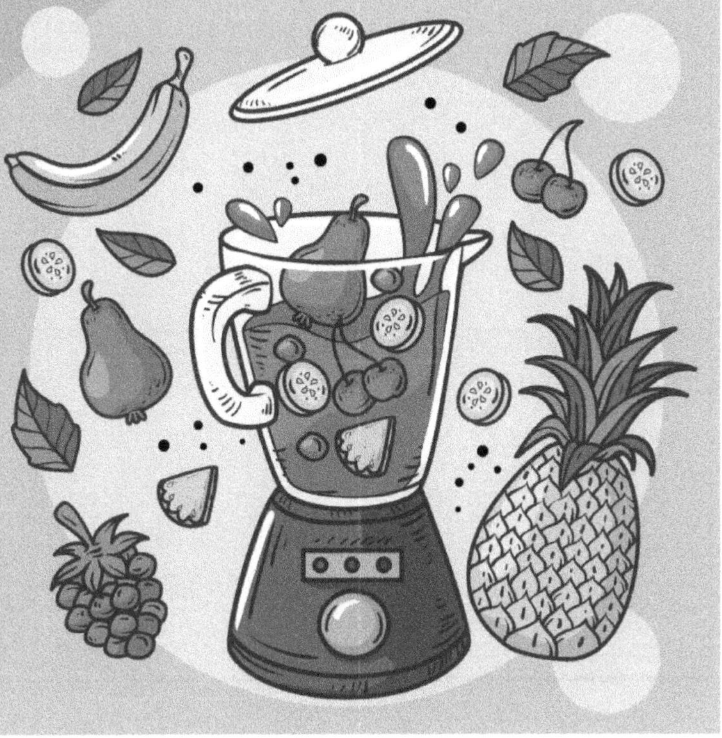

THIS BOOK BELONGS TO

Delicious Anti-Cancer Smoothies

====================================

Fight Cancer and Help Prevent Recurrence with These Easy Smoothies

---

AS Publishing

PUBLISHING

Published by **AS Publishing**

Follow Us to Stay Updated on New Releases

We offer our eBooks for free during the initial launch period. By following us, you will be among the first to know when a new eBook is released and have the opportunity to download it completely free of charge.

Don't miss out on our latest releases! Simply click on the link below, follow us, and stay up-to-date on all of our new eBooks.

amazon.com/author/as-publishing

Attribution: The resources utilized to design this cover were obtained from Pxhere.com.

Disclaimer

This book's instructions, recommendations, or methods are not intended to replace professional medical guidance, diagnosis, or care. The information in this book is only meant to be used for educational purposes; it should not be used as a replacement for professional medical advice from a healthcare provider.

The authors and publisher of this book disclaim any responsibility for any negative effects or outcomes attributable to the use of the knowledge, suggestions, or methods offered in this book. Readers should speak with their doctor before beginning any new health or wellness program.

Despite the fact that the knowledge and research upon which the information in this book is based is up-to-date, medical procedures and recommendations may alter over time.

It is advised that readers seek out additional information and keep current with healthcare trends.

The authors' views are the only ones that are expressed in this book; they do not necessarily represent the publisher's views. The authors and publisher do not endorse or recommend any companies, items, or services that are mentioned in this book.

Despite making every effort to ensure the accuracy and comprehensiveness of the information in this book, the authors and publisher make no promises or representations of any kind, either explicitly or implicitly, regarding the information's suitability, reliability, or availability.

Any risks associated with relying on the information in this book are assumed by the reader.

ISBN: 9798397467841

Contents

➢ **COMMON QUESTIONS REGARDING ANTI-CANCER SMOOTHIES9**

➢ **THE SCIENCE BEHIND ANTI-CANCER SMOOTHIES....................12**

➢ **PRACTICAL TIPS FOR INCORPORATING ANTI-CANCER SMOOTHIES INTO DAILY ROUTINES. 14**

➢ **RECIPES FOR ANTI-CANCER SMOOTHIES................................18**

❖ GREEN MACHINE DETOX SMOOTHIE INGREDIENTS: 18
❖ BERRY BLAST IMMUNITY BOOSTER INGREDIENTS:.............19
❖ TURMERIC SPICE ANTI-INFLAMMATORY SMOOTHIE INGREDIENTS:........20
❖ IMMUNE-BOOSTING CITRUS SMOOTHIE INGREDIENTS:.....................21
❖ LEAFY GREEN ANTIOXIDANT SMOOTHIE INGREDIENTS: 23
❖ GINGER-TURMERIC ANTI-INFLAMMATORY SMOOTHIE INGREDIENTS: 24
❖ BEET-BERRY ANTIOXIDANT SMOOTHIE INGREDIENTS: 25
❖ CRUCIFEROUS POWERHOUSE SMOOTHIE INGREDIENTS:.....................26
❖ CARROT-ORANGE ANTIOXIDANT SMOOTHIE INGREDIENTS: 28
❖ MORINGA-GREEN ENERGIZING SMOOTHIE INGREDIENTS: 29
❖ BLUEBERRY-GINGER ANTIOXIDANT SMOOTHIE INGREDIENTS: 30
❖ BERRY-OATMEAL BREAKFAST SMOOTHIE INGREDIENTS: 32
❖ PAPAYA-TURMERIC DIGESTIVE SMOOTHIE INGREDIENTS:.....................33
❖ PINEAPPLE-TURMERIC ANTI-INFLAMMATORY SMOOTHIE INGREDIENTS: 34
❖ MATCHA-GREEN TEA DETOX SMOOTHIE INGREDIENTS:.....................35
❖ AVOCADO-KALE POWER SMOOTHIE INGREDIENTS:............................36
❖ POMEGRANATE-BERRY IMMUNITY BOOSTING SMOOTHIE INGREDIENTS:38
❖ GINGER-TURMERIC DIGESTIVE SOOTHER INGREDIENTS:.....................39
❖ SPINACH-BERRY ANTIOXIDANT BLAST INGREDIENTS:..........................40
❖ BEETROOT-CARROT BLOOD CLEANSING SMOOTHIE INGREDIENTS:........42
❖ MANGO-TURMERIC IMMUNITY BOOSTER INGREDIENTS:.....................43
❖ BLUEBERRY-AVOCADO BRAIN BOOSTER INGREDIENTS:.......................44
❖ KALE-PINEAPPLE DIGESTIVE DETOX INGREDIENTS:...........................46
❖ TURMERIC-GREEN TEA ANTIOXIDANT ELIXIR INGREDIENTS:.................47
❖ CITRUS-CARROT VITAMIN C BOOSTER INGREDIENTS: 48
❖ BERRY-FLAXSEED OMEGA-3 BLAST INGREDIENTS: 49
❖ PINEAPPLE-CUCUMBER HYDRATION REFRESHER INGREDIENTS: 51
❖ SPINACH-AVOCADO POWERHOUSE SMOOTHIE INGREDIENTS:..............52
❖ WATERMELON-MINT COOLING REFRESHER INGREDIENTS:....................53
❖ BEETROOT-CARROT DETOX ELIXIR INGREDIENTS: 54

❖ MANGO-COCONUT ANTIOXIDANT DELIGHT INGREDIENTS: 56
❖ BLUEBERRY-WALNUT BRAIN BOOSTER INGREDIENTS: 57
❖ KALE-PINEAPPLE DIGESTIVE CLEANSE INGREDIENTS: 58
❖ TURMERIC-GINGER IMMUNE BOOSTER INGREDIENTS: 59
❖ PAPAYA-MINT DIGESTIVE SOOTHER INGREDIENTS: 61
❖ MATCHA-GREEN TEA ANTIOXIDANT BOOST INGREDIENTS: 62
❖ TOMATO-BASIL CANCER-FIGHTING ELIXIR INGREDIENTS: 63
❖ AVOCADO-SPINACH SUPERFOOD BLEND INGREDIENTS: 65
❖ RASPBERRY-BROCCOLI ANTIOXIDANT BLAST INGREDIENTS: 66
❖ MANGO-TURMERIC ENERGIZING BLEND INGREDIENTS: 67
❖ POMEGRANATE-BERRY ANTIOXIDANT BURST INGREDIENTS: 69
❖ BLUEBERRY-SPINACH BRAIN BOOSTER INGREDIENTS: 70
❖ BEETROOT-CARROT BLOOD CLEANSER INGREDIENTS: 71
❖ GINGER-TURMERIC IMMUNE BOOSTER INGREDIENTS: 72
❖ KALE-AVOCADO DETOX BLEND INGREDIENTS: 74
❖ PINEAPPLE-GREEN TEA ANTIOXIDANT BOOST INGREDIENTS: 75
❖ CHERRY-WALNUT RECOVERY BLEND INGREDIENTS: 77
❖ MANGO-CARROT GLOW BOOSTER INGREDIENTS: 78

➢ Common Questions Regarding Anti-Cancer Smoothies

1. **Are anti-cancer smoothies a substitute for medical treatment?**

   Anti-cancer smoothies should not be considered a substitute for medical treatment. While these smoothies can provide additional nutrition and support overall health, they are not a cure for cancer. It is important to consult with healthcare professionals and follow their recommended treatment plans.

2. **Can anti-cancer smoothies prevent cancer?**

   While certain foods and ingredients found in anti-cancer smoothies may have cancer-fighting properties, it is important to remember that no single food or smoothie can guarantee the prevention of cancer. A healthy diet rich in fruits, vegetables, and other nutrient-dense foods can contribute to overall health and reduce the risk of certain types of cancer, but it should be part of a comprehensive lifestyle approach to cancer prevention.

3. **Can anti-cancer smoothies cure cancer?**

   There is no scientific evidence to support the claim that anti-cancer smoothies alone can cure cancer. Cancer treatment requires a multidisciplinary approach, including medical interventions such as chemotherapy, radiation, or surgery. However, consuming a nutrient-rich diet that includes anti-cancer smoothies can support overall health and well-being during cancer treatment.

4. **Can anti-cancer smoothies interact with cancer medications?**

Some ingredients in anti-cancer smoothies, such as grapefruit or certain herbal supplements, can potentially interact with specific cancer medications. It is crucial to consult with a healthcare professional, such as an oncologist or registered dietitian, to ensure that the ingredients in your smoothies do not interfere with your medications or treatment plan.

5. **Can anti-cancer smoothies be beneficial for cancer patients?**

Anti-cancer smoothies can provide additional nutrients and hydration for cancer patients, especially those experiencing side effects from treatments like chemotherapy or radiation. However, individual dietary needs and tolerances may vary, so it is important to work with a healthcare professional to tailor smoothie recipes to specific dietary requirements and preferences.

6. **Can anti-cancer smoothies aid in recovery after cancer treatment?**

After completing cancer treatment, consuming a balanced diet that includes nutrient-dense foods like anti-cancer smoothies can support the recovery process. Smoothies can provide hydration, vitamins, minerals, and antioxidants that help replenish the body's nutrient stores. However, it is crucial to maintain a well-rounded diet and consult with a healthcare professional to ensure appropriate nutrition during the recovery phase.

7. **Can anti-cancer smoothies be enjoyed by everyone?**

Anti-cancer smoothies can be enjoyed by individuals who want to enhance their overall health and incorporate cancer-fighting ingredients into their diet. However, it is important to consider individual dietary restrictions, allergies, and health conditions. Some ingredients may not be suitable for certain individuals, so it is advisable to personalize recipes and consult with a healthcare professional or registered dietitian for personalized guidance.

Remember, maintaining a healthy lifestyle, including regular exercise, stress management, and a well-balanced diet, is key to supporting overall health and reducing the risk of chronic diseases, including cancer. Anti-cancer smoothies can be a delicious and nutritious addition to a healthy diet, but they should be part of a comprehensive approach to cancer prevention and treatment.

➢ **The Science Behind Anti-Cancer Smoothies**

Anti-cancer smoothies are often based on scientific evidence regarding the potential health benefits of specific ingredients. While it's important to note that these smoothies are not a cure for cancer and should not replace medical treatment, they can be a part of a well-rounded, nutritious diet that supports overall health and potentially reduces the risk of cancer. Here are some key scientific considerations behind anti-cancer smoothies:

1. **Antioxidants:** Many anti-cancer smoothie recipes emphasize ingredients rich in antioxidants. Antioxidants are compounds that help protect cells from damage caused by free radicals, unstable molecules that can lead to cellular damage and increase the risk of cancer. Fruits and vegetables, such as berries, citrus fruits, leafy greens, and deeply colored produce, are often included in anti-cancer smoothies due to their high antioxidant content.

2. **Phytochemicals:** Phytochemicals are naturally occurring compounds found in plants that have been associated with various health benefits, including cancer prevention. Examples of phytochemicals found in anti-cancer smoothie ingredients include carotenoids (e.g., beta-carotene in carrots), flavonoids (e.g., quercetin in berries), and glucosinolates (e.g., sulforaphane in cruciferous vegetables). These phytochemicals have been studied for their potential to inhibit cancer cell growth and reduce inflammation.

3. **Fiber:** Many anti-cancer smoothie recipes incorporate ingredients high in dietary fiber, such as fruits, vegetables, whole grains, and seeds. Adequate fiber intake is associated with a lower risk of colorectal cancer. Fiber helps maintain regular bowel movements, aids in digestion, and may contribute to a healthier gut microbiome, which plays a role in overall health and disease prevention.

4. **Healthy Fats:** Some anti-cancer smoothies include ingredients rich in healthy fats, such as avocado, nuts, and seeds. These fats provide essential fatty acids and are sources of antioxidants, which can have anti-inflammatory effects. Omega-3 fatty acids, in particular, found in ingredients like flaxseeds and chia seeds, have been studied for their potential anti-cancer properties.

5. **Hydration:** Many anti-cancer smoothies include hydrating ingredients, such as coconut water or water-based fruits and vegetables. Staying adequately hydrated is essential for overall health, including maintaining proper bodily functions and supporting cellular health.

6. **Overall Nutrient Density:** Anti-cancer smoothies are often designed to be nutrient-dense, incorporating a variety of fruits, vegetables, nuts, seeds, and other ingredients rich in vitamins, minerals, and phytochemicals. A diet rich in nutrient-dense foods supports overall health and provides the body with the necessary tools to

maintain proper functioning and potentially reduce the risk of cancer.

It's important to note that while specific ingredients in anti-cancer smoothies may have scientific support for their potential health benefits, the overall impact on cancer prevention is influenced by various factors, including genetics, lifestyle, and environmental factors. Additionally, it's crucial to consult with healthcare professionals or registered dietitians to tailor dietary choices to individual needs and to ensure that anti-cancer smoothies complement a comprehensive approach to cancer prevention and treatment.

➤ Practical tips for incorporating anti-cancer smoothies into daily routines.

Incorporating anti-cancer smoothies into your daily routine can be a delicious and convenient way to boost your nutrient intake and support overall health. Here are some practical tips to help you seamlessly integrate anti-cancer smoothies into your lifestyle:

1. **Plan Ahead:** Take a few minutes each week to plan your smoothie recipes and create a shopping list. This will ensure you have all the necessary ingredients on hand and can easily prepare your smoothies without last-minute trips to the grocery store.

2. **Prep Ingredients in Advance:** Save time in the mornings by prepping some ingredients in advance. Wash and chop fruits and vegetables, portion out ingredients, and freeze them if needed. This way, you can quickly grab and blend the ingredients without the hassle of prep work.

3. **Invest in a High-Quality Blender:** A powerful blender can make a significant difference in the texture and consistency of your smoothies. Invest in a blender that can handle frozen fruits, leafy greens, and nuts to create smooth and well-blended concoctions.

4. **Experiment with Flavors and Ingredients:** Don't be afraid to get creative and experiment with different flavors and ingredients. Mix and match fruits, vegetables, herbs, and spices to find your favorite combinations. This will help keep your smoothies exciting and enjoyable.

5. **Consider Nutritional Balance:** Aim for a balance of macronutrients in your smoothies. Include a source of protein, such as Greek yogurt, silken tofu, or plant-based protein powder, to help keep you satiated. Add healthy fats from ingredients like avocado, nuts, or seeds to promote nutrient absorption and provide a feeling of fullness.

6. **Customize to Your Taste:** Adjust the sweetness, thickness, and consistency of your smoothies to your liking. You can add natural sweeteners like honey, maple syrup, or dates if desired. If you prefer a thicker smoothie, add ice cubes or frozen

fruits. If you like a thinner consistency, increase the liquid content.

7. **Make it a Meal:** If you're using smoothies as a meal replacement or a substantial snack, consider adding additional ingredients to make them more satisfying and nutritionally balanced. You can incorporate oats, nut butter, chia seeds, or even leafy greens to boost the nutritional content and make the smoothie more filling.

8. **Enjoy at Any Time:** While smoothies are commonly associated with breakfast, they can be enjoyed at any time of the day. Have a smoothie as a refreshing midday snack, post-workout replenishment, or even a healthy dessert option.

9. **Involve the Whole Family:** Get your family involved in the smoothie-making process. Let children help choose ingredients and assist in blending. This can make it a fun and interactive activity while encouraging them to consume more fruits and vegetables.

10. **Variety is Key:** Don't limit yourself to just one or two smoothie recipes. Explore a variety of anti-cancer smoothie recipes to keep things interesting and ensure you benefit from a wide range of nutrients. Rotate your ingredients and experiment with new flavors to avoid taste fatigue.

Remember, while anti-cancer smoothies can be a valuable addition to a healthy lifestyle, they should not replace a well-balanced diet. It's important to consume a variety of whole foods, including fruits, vegetables, whole grains, lean proteins, and healthy fats, alongside your smoothies to provide a comprehensive and balanced nutritional intake.

Consult with healthcare professionals or registered dietitians for personalized advice and guidance, especially if you have specific dietary needs or health concerns. Enjoy the process of creating and savoring your anti-cancer smoothies as part of a holistic approach to overall well-being.

➢ Recipes for Anti-Cancer Smoothies

❖ Green Machine Detox Smoothie Ingredients:

- 1 cup spinach (rich in antioxidants and chlorophyll)
- 1 cucumber (hydrating and supports detoxification)
- 1 green apple (high in fiber and phytochemicals)
- 1/2 lemon, juiced (packed with vitamin C)
- 1-inch piece of ginger (anti-inflammatory and aids digestion)
- 1 cup coconut water (rich in electrolytes)

Instructions:

1. Wash the spinach, cucumber, and apple thoroughly.
2. Peel the cucumber and chop it into small pieces.
3. Core the apple and cut it into chunks.
4. Add all the ingredients to a blender.
5. Blend until smooth and creamy.
6. If desired, add ice cubes for a refreshing chill.
7. Pour into a glass and enjoy immediately.

Benefits: This smoothie provides a powerful detoxification boost, thanks to the combination of spinach, cucumber, and lemon. The antioxidants present in spinach help neutralize harmful free radicals, while cucumber hydrates the body and aids in flushing out toxins. The ginger and lemon juice contribute to the smoothie's cleansing properties.

❖ Berry Blast Immunity Booster Ingredients:

- 1 cup mixed berries (blueberries, strawberries, raspberries)

- 1 small banana (aids digestion and adds creaminess)

- 1 cup almond milk (contains vitamin E and healthy fats)

- 1 tablespoon chia seeds (packed with omega-3 fatty acids)

- 1 tablespoon honey or maple syrup (optional for added sweetness)

Instructions:

1. Wash the berries thoroughly.

2. Peel and slice the banana.

3. Add the berries, banana, almond milk, chia seeds, and sweetener (if using) to a blender.

4. Blend until smooth and creamy.

5. Taste and adjust sweetness if needed.

6. Pour into a glass and serve immediately.

Benefits: Berries are known for their high antioxidant content, which helps protect cells from damage and reduce the risk of cancer. The combination of berries, banana, and chia seeds provides a rich source of vitamins, minerals, and fiber. The almond milk adds creaminess and contributes healthy fats.

❖ Turmeric Spice Anti-Inflammatory Smoothie Ingredients:

- 1 cup coconut milk (contains medium-chain triglycerides)

- 1 small ripe mango (rich in vitamins A and C)

- 1 teaspoon turmeric powder (potent anti-inflammatory properties)

- 1/2 teaspoon cinnamon (supports blood sugar balance)

- 1 tablespoon flaxseeds (source of omega-3 fatty acids)

- 1 tablespoon almond butter (adds creaminess and healthy fats)

- 1 teaspoon honey or maple syrup (optional for added sweetness)

Instructions:

1. Peel and chop the mango into small pieces.

2. Add the mango, coconut milk, turmeric powder, cinnamon, flaxseeds, almond butter, and sweetener (if using) to a blender.

3. Blend until smooth and creamy.

4. Taste and adjust sweetness if needed.

5. Pour into a glass and enjoy immediately.

Benefits: Turmeric is a powerful anti-inflammatory spice that has been shown to inhibit the growth of cancer cells. Mango and cinnamon both possess antioxidant properties, while flaxseeds provide omega-3 fatty acids that support overall health. The almond butter adds a creamy texture and healthy fats.

❖ **Immune-Boosting Citrus Smoothie**
   Ingredients:

- 1 large orange (high in vitamin C and antioxidants)

- 1 small grapefruit (rich in lycopene and vitamin A)

- 1 cup pineapple chunks (contains bromelain, which aids digestion)

- 1/2 cup Greek yogurt (provides probiotics and protein)

- 1 tablespoon honey or agave syrup (optional for added sweetness)

- Ice cubes (optional)

Instructions:

1. Peel the orange and grapefruit, removing any seeds.

2. Cut the citrus fruits into segments.

3. Add the orange segments, grapefruit segments, pineapple chunks, Greek yogurt, and sweetener (if using) to a blender.

4. Blend until smooth and creamy.

5. If desired, add ice cubes for a refreshing chill.

6. Pour into a glass and enjoy immediately.

Benefits: This smoothie is packed with immune-boosting properties from the citrus fruits, which are rich in vitamin C and antioxidants. Pineapple adds digestive benefits due to the enzyme bromelain, while Greek yogurt provides probiotics that support a healthy gut. The optional honey or agave syrup adds natural sweetness.

❖ Leafy Green Antioxidant Smoothie
Ingredients:

- 2 cups kale or spinach (loaded with antioxidants and chlorophyll)

- 1 cup fresh or frozen berries (such as blueberries or raspberries)

- 1 small avocado (provides healthy fats and creaminess)

- 1 tablespoon hemp seeds (source of omega-3 fatty acids and protein)

- 1 cup unsweetened almond milk (or other plant-based milk)

- 1 tablespoon lime juice (rich in vitamin C)

- Ice cubes (optional)

Instructions:

1. Wash the kale or spinach leaves thoroughly.

2. Remove the stems and tear the leaves into smaller pieces.

3. Add the kale or spinach, berries, avocado, hemp seeds, almond milk, lime juice, and ice cubes (if using) to a blender.

4. Blend until smooth and creamy.

5. Pour into a glass and serve immediately.

Benefits: This smoothie is a powerhouse of antioxidants from the leafy greens and berries, which help protect cells from damage. Avocado adds healthy fats and creaminess, while hemp seeds provide omega-3 fatty acids and protein. Lime juice adds a refreshing citrus kick.

❖ **Ginger-Turmeric Anti-Inflammatory Smoothie**
Ingredients:

- 1 cup coconut water (hydrating and rich in electrolytes)

- 1 small ripe banana (adds creaminess and potassium)

- 1-inch piece of ginger root (anti-inflammatory and aids digestion)

- 1 teaspoon turmeric powder (potent anti-inflammatory properties)

- 1 tablespoon almond butter (provides healthy fats and creaminess)

- 1 tablespoon chia seeds (packed with omega-3 fatty acids)

- 1 tablespoon honey or maple syrup (optional for added sweetness)

Instructions:

1. Peel and slice the ginger root.

2. Add the coconut water, banana, ginger root, turmeric powder, almond butter, chia seeds, and sweetener (if using) to a blender.

3. Blend until smooth and creamy.

4. Taste and adjust sweetness if needed.

5. Pour into a glass and enjoy immediately.

Benefits: This smoothie combines the anti-inflammatory powers of ginger and turmeric to help reduce inflammation in the body. Coconut water provides hydration and electrolytes, while banana adds potassium. The almond butter and chia seeds contribute healthy fats and omega-3 fatty acids.

❖ Beet-Berry Antioxidant Smoothie Ingredients:

- 1 small cooked beetroot (high in antioxidants and nitrates)

- 1 cup mixed berries (such as strawberries, blueberries, and raspberries)

- 1 small apple (rich in fiber and phytochemicals)

- 1 cup almond milk (or other plant-based milk)

- 1 tablespoon honey or agave syrup (optional for added sweetness)

- Ice cubes (optional)

Instructions:

1. Peel and chop the cooked beetroot into small pieces.

2. Wash the berries and apple thoroughly.

3. Core the apple and cut it into chunks.

4. Add the beetroot, berries, apple chunks, almond milk, and sweetener (if using) to a blender.

5. Blend until smooth and well combined.

6. If desired, add ice cubes for a refreshing chill.

7. Pour into a glass and serve immediately.

Benefits: This vibrant smoothie is packed with antioxidants from the beetroot and mixed berries, which help combat oxidative stress. The apple adds fiber and additional antioxidants, while almond milk provides a creamy base. The optional honey or agave syrup adds natural sweetness.

❖ **Cruciferous Powerhouse Smoothie**
   Ingredients:

- 1 cup kale (rich in antioxidants and fiber)

- 1 cup broccoli florets (contains sulforaphane, a cancer-fighting compound)

- 1/2 cup pineapple chunks (adds sweetness and bromelain)

- 1 small banana (provides creaminess and potassium)

- 1 tablespoon flaxseeds (source of omega-3 fatty acids)

- 1 cup coconut water (hydrating and rich in electrolytes)

- Ice cubes (optional)

Instructions:

1. Wash the kale thoroughly and remove the stems.

2. Cut the broccoli florets into smaller pieces.

3. Add the kale, broccoli, pineapple chunks, banana, flaxseeds, coconut water, and ice cubes (if using) to a blender.

4. Blend until smooth and creamy.

5. Pour into a glass and enjoy immediately.

Benefits: This smoothie harnesses the power of cruciferous vegetables like kale and broccoli, which are rich in antioxidants and contain compounds that support cancer prevention. Pineapple adds natural sweetness and bromelain, while the banana provides creaminess and potassium. Flaxseeds contribute omega-3 fatty acids for added health benefits.

❖ **Carrot-Orange Antioxidant Smoothie**
   Ingredients:

- 2 medium carrots (high in beta-carotene and antioxidants)
- 1 large orange (packed with vitamin C and folate)
- 1 small apple (rich in fiber and phytochemicals)
- 1 tablespoon fresh lemon juice (provides vitamin C)
- 1/2 cup coconut water (hydrating and rich in electrolytes)
- 1 tablespoon honey or maple syrup (optional for added sweetness)
- Ice cubes (optional)

Instructions:

1. Peel and chop the carrots into small pieces.
2. Peel the orange, removing any seeds.
3. Core the apple and cut it into chunks.
4. Add the carrots, orange segments, apple chunks, lemon juice, coconut water, and sweetener (if using) to a blender.

5. Blend until smooth and well combined.

6. If desired, add ice cubes for a refreshing chill.

7. Pour into a glass and serve immediately.

Benefits: This vibrant smoothie is bursting with antioxidants from the carrots, orange, and apple. Carrots are particularly rich in beta-carotene, which supports immune function and skin health. The lemon juice adds a tangy flavor and vitamin C, while coconut water provides hydration and electrolytes.

❖ **Moringa-Green Energizing Smoothie**
   Ingredients:

- 1 cup spinach (packed with antioxidants and iron)

- 1 ripe banana (provides energy and potassium)

- 1 tablespoon moringa powder (rich in nutrients and antioxidants)

- 1 tablespoon almond butter (adds creaminess and healthy fats)

- 1 cup almond milk (or other plant-based milk)

- 1 tablespoon honey or maple syrup (optional for added sweetness)

- Ice cubes (optional)

Instructions:

1. Wash the spinach leaves thoroughly.

2. Peel and slice the ripe banana.

3. Add the spinach, banana slices, moringa powder, almond butter, almond milk, and sweetener (if using) to a blender.

4. Blend until smooth and creamy.

5. If desired, add ice cubes for a refreshing chill.

6. Pour into a glass and enjoy immediately.

Benefits: This energizing smoothie combines the nutritional power of spinach and moringa powder. Spinach is rich in antioxidants and iron, providing a boost of energy. Moringa powder offers a range of nutrients and antioxidants that support overall health. The banana adds natural sweetness and potassium, while almond butter contributes healthy fats.

❖ **Blueberry-Ginger Antioxidant Smoothie Ingredients:**

- 1 cup blueberries (loaded with antioxidants and phytochemicals)

- 1 small ripe pear (rich in fiber and vitamin C)

- 1-inch piece of ginger root (anti-inflammatory and aids digestion)

- 1 tablespoon flaxseeds (source of omega-3 fatty acids)

- 1 cup coconut water (hydrating and rich in electrolytes)

- 1 tablespoon honey or agave syrup (optional for added sweetness)

- Ice cubes (optional)

Instructions:

1. Wash the blueberries and pear thoroughly.

2. Core the pear and cut it into chunks.

3. Peel and slice the ginger root.

4. Add the blueberries, pear chunks, ginger root, flaxseeds, coconut water, and sweetener (if using) to a blender.

5. Blend until smooth and well combined.

6. If desired, add ice cubes for a refreshing chill.

7. Pour into a glass and serve immediately.

Benefits: Blueberries are known for their high antioxidant content, which helps protect cells from damage. The ginger root adds a zesty kick and contributes to the smoothie's anti-inflammatory properties. The pear provides fiber and vitamin C, while flaxseeds offer omega-

3 fatty acids. Coconut water hydrates the body and adds electrolytes.

❖ **Berry-Oatmeal Breakfast Smoothie**
   Ingredients:

- 1 cup mixed berries (such as strawberries, blueberries, and raspberries)

- 1/2 cup rolled oats (high in fiber and provide sustained energy)

- 1 tablespoon almond butter (adds creaminess and healthy fats)

- 1 cup almond milk (or other plant-based milk)

- 1 tablespoon honey or maple syrup (optional for added sweetness)

- Ice cubes (optional)

Instructions:

1. Wash the berries thoroughly.

2. Add the mixed berries, rolled oats, almond butter, almond milk, and sweetener (if using) to a blender.

3. Blend until smooth and well combined.

4. If desired, add ice cubes for a refreshing chill.

5. Pour into a glass and enjoy immediately.

Benefits: This smoothie combines the goodness of mixed berries and oats. Berries are rich in antioxidants and fiber, while oats provide sustained energy and promote a feeling of fullness. The almond butter adds creaminess and healthy fats, and the almond milk creates a smooth texture.

❖ **Papaya-Turmeric Digestive Smoothie
   Ingredients:**

- 1 cup ripe papaya chunks (rich in digestive enzymes and antioxidants)

- 1 small banana (provides creaminess and potassium)

- 1 teaspoon turmeric powder (anti-inflammatory and aids digestion)

- 1/2 cup Greek yogurt (provides probiotics and protein)

- 1 tablespoon chia seeds (packed with fiber and omega-3 fatty acids)

- 1 cup coconut water (hydrating and rich in electrolytes)

- Ice cubes (optional)

Instructions:

1. Peel and cut the papaya into chunks.

2. Peel the banana and slice it.

3. Add the papaya chunks, banana slices, turmeric powder, Greek yogurt, chia seeds, coconut water, and ice cubes (if using) to a blender.

4. Blend until smooth and creamy.

5. Pour into a glass and serve immediately.

Benefits: Papaya contains digestive enzymes that aid in the breakdown of food and promote healthy digestion. Turmeric contributes anti-inflammatory properties, while the banana adds creaminess and potassium. Greek yogurt provides probiotics for gut health, and chia seeds offer fiber and omega-3 fatty acids.

❖ Pineapple-Turmeric Anti-Inflammatory Smoothie Ingredients:

- 1 cup pineapple chunks (contains bromelain, which aids digestion)

- 1 small ripe banana (provides creaminess and potassium)

- 1 teaspoon turmeric powder (potent anti-inflammatory properties)

- 1 tablespoon coconut oil (provides healthy fats)

- 1 cup coconut water (hydrating and rich in electrolytes)

- 1 tablespoon honey or maple syrup (optional for added sweetness)

- Ice cubes (optional)

Instructions:

1. Add the pineapple chunks, banana, turmeric powder, coconut oil, coconut water, and sweetener (if using) to a blender.

2. Blend until smooth and creamy.

3. If desired, add ice cubes for a refreshing chill.

4. Pour into a glass and enjoy immediately.

Benefits: This tropical smoothie combines the anti-inflammatory properties of turmeric with the digestion-enhancing benefits of pineapple. The banana adds creaminess and potassium, while coconut oil provides healthy fats. Coconut water keeps you hydrated, and the optional sweetener adds a touch of sweetness.

❖ **Matcha-Green Tea Detox Smoothie**
   Ingredients:

- 1 cup unsweetened almond milk (or other plant-based milk)

- 1 teaspoon matcha powder (loaded with antioxidants)

- 1/2 teaspoon spirulina powder (detoxifying and nutrient-rich)

- 1 tablespoon almond butter (adds creaminess and healthy fats)

- 1 tablespoon honey or agave syrup (optional for added sweetness)

- Ice cubes (optional)

Instructions:

1. Add the almond milk, matcha powder, spirulina powder, almond butter, and sweetener (if using) to a blender.

2. Blend until well combined.

3. If desired, add ice cubes for a refreshing chill.

4. Pour into a glass and enjoy immediately.

Benefits: This vibrant green smoothie combines the antioxidant power of matcha with the detoxifying properties of spirulina. Almond butter adds creaminess and healthy fats, while almond milk provides a smooth base. The optional sweetener enhances the flavor profile.

❖ Avocado-Kale Power Smoothie Ingredients:

- 1 cup kale leaves (rich in antioxidants and fiber)

- 1/2 ripe avocado (packed with healthy fats and vitamins)

- 1 small ripe banana (provides creaminess and potassium)

- 1 tablespoon almond butter (adds additional creaminess and healthy fats)

- 1 cup almond milk (or other plant-based milk)

- 1 tablespoon honey or maple syrup (optional for added sweetness)

- Ice cubes (optional)

Instructions:

1. Wash the kale leaves thoroughly and remove the stems.

2. Scoop out the flesh of the avocado.

3. Add the kale leaves, avocado, banana, almond butter, almond milk, and sweetener (if using) to a blender.

4. Blend until smooth and creamy.

5. If desired, add ice cubes for a refreshing chill.

6. Pour into a glass and enjoy immediately.

Benefits: This power-packed smoothie combines the nutritional benefits of kale and avocado. Kale is rich in antioxidants and fiber, while avocado provides healthy fats and essential vitamins. The banana adds creaminess and potassium, and almond butter contributes to the smoothie's creamy texture and healthy fats.

❖ Pomegranate-Berry Immunity Boosting Smoothie Ingredients:

- 1 cup pomegranate juice (high in antioxidants and immune-boosting properties)

- 1 cup mixed berries (such as strawberries, blueberries, and raspberries)

- 1 small ripe banana (provides creaminess and potassium)

- 1 tablespoon flaxseeds (source of omega-3 fatty acids)

- 1/2 cup Greek yogurt (provides probiotics and protein)

- Ice cubes (optional)

Instructions:

1. Add the pomegranate juice, mixed berries, banana, flaxseeds, and Greek yogurt to a blender.

2. Blend until smooth and well combined.

3. If desired, add ice cubes for a refreshing chill.

4. Pour into a glass and serve immediately.

Benefits: This smoothie is packed with immune-boosting ingredients. Pomegranate juice is rich in antioxidants that help support a healthy immune system. Mixed berries provide additional antioxidants, while the banana adds creaminess and potassium. Flaxseeds contribute omega-3 fatty acids, and Greek yogurt offers probiotics and protein.

❖ **Ginger-Turmeric Digestive Soother**
   Ingredients:

- 1 cup unsweetened coconut milk (or other plant-based milk)

- 1-inch piece of ginger root (anti-inflammatory and aids digestion)

- 1 teaspoon turmeric powder (potent anti-inflammatory properties)

- 1 tablespoon honey or maple syrup (optional for added sweetness)

- 1/2 teaspoon vanilla extract (optional for flavor)

- Pinch of black pepper (increases turmeric absorption)

- Ice cubes (optional)

Instructions:

1. Peel and slice the ginger root.

2. Add the coconut milk, ginger slices, turmeric powder, sweetener (if using), vanilla extract, and black pepper to a blender.

3. Blend until well combined.

4. If desired, add ice cubes for a refreshing chill.

5. Pour into a glass and enjoy immediately.

Benefits: This soothing smoothie combines the digestive benefits of ginger and the anti-inflammatory properties of turmeric. Ginger helps ease digestion and reduce inflammation, while turmeric provides potent anti-inflammatory compounds. The coconut milk adds creaminess, and the optional sweetener and vanilla extract enhance the flavor.

❖ Spinach-Berry Antioxidant Blast Ingredients:

- 1 cup spinach leaves (packed with antioxidants and iron)

- 1 cup mixed berries (such as strawberries, blueberries, and raspberries)

- 1 small ripe banana (provides creaminess and potassium)

- 1 tablespoon almond butter (adds creaminess and healthy fats)

- 1 cup almond milk (or other plant-based milk)

- 1 tablespoon honey or maple syrup (optional for added sweetness)

- Ice cubes (optional)

Instructions:

1. Wash the spinach leaves thoroughly.

2. Add the spinach, mixed berries, banana, almond butter, almond milk, and sweetener (if using) to a blender.

3. Blend until smooth and well combined.

4. If desired, add ice cubes for a refreshing chill.

5. Pour into a glass and enjoy immediately.

Benefits: This antioxidant-rich smoothie combines the nutritional power of spinach and mixed berries. Spinach is loaded with antioxidants and iron, while the mixed berries provide additional antioxidants and a burst of natural sweetness. The banana adds creaminess and potassium, and almond butter contributes to the smoothie's texture and healthy fats.

❖ Beetroot-Carrot Blood Cleansing Smoothie
Ingredients:

- 1 medium-sized beetroot (rich in antioxidants and supports detoxification)

- 2 medium-sized carrots (high in beta-carotene and vitamin A)

- 1 small apple (adds natural sweetness and fiber)

- 1-inch piece of ginger root (anti-inflammatory and aids digestion)

- 1 cup coconut water (hydrating and rich in electrolytes)

- 1 tablespoon lemon juice (cleansing and alkalizing)

- Ice cubes (optional)

Instructions:

1. Wash the beetroot, carrots, apple, and ginger root thoroughly.

2. Peel the beetroot, carrots, and ginger root.

3. Cut the beetroot, carrots, and apple into small chunks.

4. Add the beetroot chunks, carrot chunks, apple chunks, ginger root, coconut water, lemon juice, and ice cubes (if using) to a blender.

5. Blend until smooth and well combined.

6. Pour into a glass and serve immediately.

Benefits: This blood-cleansing smoothie harnesses the power of beetroot, carrots, and ginger root. Beetroot is rich in antioxidants and supports detoxification processes in the body. Carrots provide beta-carotene and vitamin A, which are beneficial for healthy blood cells. Ginger root aids digestion and adds a zesty kick, while the apple contributes natural sweetness and fiber. Coconut water hydrates the body, and lemon juice provides cleansing and alkalizing properties.

❖ **Mango-Turmeric Immunity Booster**
 Ingredients:

- 1 cup ripe mango chunks (packed with vitamin C and antioxidants)

- 1 small ripe banana (provides creaminess and potassium)

- 1 teaspoon turmeric powder (potent anti-inflammatory properties)

- 1 tablespoon hemp seeds (rich in omega-3 fatty acids and protein)

- 1 cup coconut milk (or other plant-based milk)

- 1 tablespoon honey or maple syrup (optional for added sweetness)

- Ice cubes (optional)

Instructions:

1. Add the mango chunks, banana, turmeric powder, hemp seeds, coconut milk, and sweetener (if using) to a blender.

2. Blend until smooth and creamy.

3. If desired, add ice cubes for a refreshing chill.

4. Pour into a glass and enjoy immediately.

Benefits: This immunity-boosting smoothie combines the tropical flavors of mango with the anti-inflammatory properties of turmeric. Mango is rich in vitamin C and antioxidants, which support a healthy immune system. The banana adds creaminess and potassium, while hemp seeds provide omega-3 fatty acids and protein. Coconut milk adds a creamy texture and healthy fats.

❖ **Blueberry-Avocado Brain Booster Ingredients:**

- 1 cup blueberries (rich in antioxidants and promote brain health)

- 1/2 ripe avocado (packed with healthy fats and vitamins)

- 1 small ripe banana (provides creaminess and potassium)

- 1 tablespoon almond butter (adds creaminess and healthy fats)

- 1 cup almond milk (or other plant-based milk)

- 1 tablespoon honey or maple syrup (optional for added sweetness)

- Ice cubes (optional)

Instructions:

1. Wash the blueberries thoroughly.

2. Cut the avocado in half and scoop out the flesh.

3. Add the blueberries, avocado, banana, almond butter, almond milk, and sweetener (if using) to a blender.

4. Blend until smooth and well combined.

5. If desired, add ice cubes for a refreshing chill.

6. Pour into a glass and enjoy immediately.

Benefits: This brain-boosting smoothie combines the antioxidant power of blueberries with the healthy fats and vitamins from avocado. Blueberries are known for their brain-enhancing properties and high levels of antioxidants. Avocado adds creaminess and provides essential nutrients and healthy fats. The banana adds potassium, almond butter contributes to the smooth texture and healthy fats, and almond milk serves as a nutritious base.

❖ Kale-Pineapple Digestive Detox Ingredients:

- 1 cup kale leaves (rich in fiber and aids digestion)

- 1 cup pineapple chunks (contains bromelain for digestion)

- 1 small cucumber (hydrating and aids detoxification)

- 1-inch piece of ginger root (anti-inflammatory and aids digestion)

- 1 tablespoon lemon juice (cleansing and alkalizing)

- 1 cup coconut water (hydrating and rich in electrolytes)

- Ice cubes (optional)

Instructions:

1. Wash the kale leaves thoroughly and remove the stems.

2. Cut the pineapple into small chunks.

3. Peel and slice the cucumber.

4. Peel the ginger root.

5. Add the kale leaves, pineapple chunks, cucumber slices, ginger root, lemon juice, coconut water, and ice cubes (if using) to a blender.

6. Blend until smooth and well combined.

7. Pour into a glass and serve immediately.

Benefits: This refreshing smoothie combines the cleansing properties of kale, pineapple, cucumber, and ginger for a digestive detox. Kale provides fiber for healthy digestion, while pineapple contains bromelain, an enzyme that aids in the breakdown of proteins. Cucumber hydrates the body and supports detoxification processes, while ginger root aids digestion and adds a zingy flavor. Lemon juice provides cleansing and alkalizing benefits, and coconut water hydrates and replenishes electrolytes.

❖ **Turmeric-Green Tea Antioxidant Elixir**
   Ingredients:

- 1 teaspoon turmeric powder (potent anti-inflammatory properties)

- 1 teaspoon matcha green tea powder (high in antioxidants)

- 1 cup unsweetened almond milk (or other plant-based milk)

- 1 tablespoon honey or maple syrup (optional for added sweetness)

- 1/2 teaspoon vanilla extract (optional for flavor)

- Ice cubes (optional)

Instructions:

1. In a small bowl, mix the turmeric powder and matcha green tea powder together.

2. In a saucepan, heat the almond milk over low heat until warm but not boiling.

3. Add the turmeric-matcha mixture to the warm almond milk and whisk until well combined.

4. Stir in the sweetener (if using) and vanilla extract.

5. If desired, transfer the mixture to a blender and blend for a few seconds to create a frothy texture.

6. Pour into a cup and serve immediately.

Benefits: This antioxidant elixir combines the anti-inflammatory properties of turmeric with the high antioxidant content of matcha green tea. Turmeric helps reduce inflammation in the body, while matcha green tea provides a boost of antioxidants. Almond milk serves as a creamy and dairy-free base, and the optional sweetener and vanilla extract add flavor to the elixir.

❖ Citrus-Carrot Vitamin C Booster Ingredients:

- 2 medium-sized oranges (high in vitamin C)

- 2 medium-sized carrots (rich in beta-carotene and vitamin A)

- 1 small lemon (cleansing and alkalizing)

- 1 small piece of ginger root (anti-inflammatory and aids digestion)

- 1 tablespoon honey or maple syrup (optional for added sweetness)

- Ice cubes (optional)

Instructions:

1. Peel the oranges and lemon, and remove the seeds.

2. Wash and peel the carrots.

3. Peel the ginger root.

4. Add the peeled oranges, carrots, lemon, ginger root, and sweetener (if using) to a blender.

5. Blend until smooth and well combined.

6. If desired, add ice cubes for a refreshing chill.

7. Pour into a glass and enjoy immediately.

Benefits: This vitamin C booster is packed with citrus fruits and carrots. Oranges and lemons are rich in vitamin C, which supports a healthy immune system. Carrots provide beta-carotene and vitamin A for overall well-being. Ginger root aids digestion and adds a zesty kick to the smoothie. The optional sweetener enhances the taste.

❖ **Berry-Flaxseed Omega-3 Blast Ingredients:**

- 1 cup mixed berries (such as strawberries, blueberries, and raspberries)
- 1 tablespoon ground flaxseeds (rich in omega-3 fatty acids)
- 1 small ripe banana (provides creaminess and potassium)
- 1 cup almond milk (or other plant-based milk)
- 1 tablespoon honey or maple syrup (optional for added sweetness)
- Ice cubes (optional)

Instructions:

1. Wash the mixed berries thoroughly.
2. Add the mixed berries, ground flaxseeds, banana, almond milk, and sweetener (if using) to a blender.
3. Blend until smooth and well combined.
4. If desired, add ice cubes for a refreshing chill.
5. Pour into a glass and enjoy immediately.

Benefits: This omega-3 blast smoothie combines the antioxidant power of mixed berries with the nutritional benefits of flaxseeds. Berries are rich in antioxidants, while flaxseeds provide essential omega-3 fatty acids for brain health and inflammation reduction. The banana adds creaminess and potassium, and almond milk serves as a nutritious base. The optional sweetener enhances the taste.

❖ **Pineapple-Cucumber Hydration Refresher**
   Ingredients:

- 1 cup pineapple chunks (contains bromelain for digestion)
- 1 small cucumber (hydrating and aids detoxification)
- 1/2 cup coconut water (hydrating and rich in electrolytes)
- 1 tablespoon lime juice (refreshing and alkalizing)
- 1 tablespoon fresh mint leaves (optional for added freshness)
- Ice cubes (optional)

Instructions:

1. Cut the pineapple into small chunks.
2. Peel and slice the cucumber.
3. Add the pineapple chunks, cucumber slices, coconut water, lime juice, fresh mint leaves (if using), and ice cubes (if using) to a blender.
4. Blend until smooth and well combined.

5. Pour into a glass and serve immediately.

Benefits: This hydration refresher combines the tropical flavors of pineapple with the hydrating properties of cucumber and coconut water. Pineapple contains bromelain, an enzyme that aids in digestion, while cucumber helps detoxify and hydrate the body. Coconut water replenishes electrolytes, and lime juice adds a refreshing zing. The fresh mint leaves provide added freshness.

❖ **Spinach-Avocado Powerhouse Smoothie Ingredients:**

- 1 cup fresh spinach leaves (packed with vitamins and minerals)

- 1/2 ripe avocado (rich in healthy fats and fiber)

- 1 small ripe banana (provides creaminess and potassium)

- 1 tablespoon almond butter (adds creaminess and healthy fats)

- 1 cup almond milk (or other plant-based milk)

- 1 tablespoon honey or maple syrup (optional for added sweetness)

- Ice cubes (optional)

Instructions:

1. Wash the spinach leaves thoroughly.

2. Cut the avocado in half and scoop out the flesh.

3. Add the spinach leaves, avocado, banana, almond butter, almond milk, and sweetener (if using) to a blender.

4. Blend until smooth and well combined.

5. If desired, add ice cubes for a refreshing chill.

6. Pour into a glass and enjoy immediately.

Benefits: This powerhouse smoothie combines the nutrient-rich spinach with the healthy fats and fiber from avocado. Spinach is packed with vitamins, minerals, and antioxidants that support overall health. Avocado adds creaminess and provides essential nutrients and healthy fats. The banana adds potassium, almond butter contributes to the smooth texture and healthy fats, and almond milk serves as a nutritious base.

❖ **Watermelon-Mint Cooling Refresher**
   Ingredients:

- 2 cups fresh watermelon chunks (hydrating and rich in antioxidants)

- 1 tablespoon lime juice (refreshing and alkalizing)

- 1 tablespoon fresh mint leaves

- Ice cubes (optional)

Instructions:

1. Cut the watermelon into small chunks, removing any seeds.

2. Add the watermelon chunks, lime juice, fresh mint leaves, and ice cubes (if using) to a blender.

3. Blend until smooth and well combined.

4. Pour into a glass and serve immediately.

Benefits: This cooling refresher combines the hydrating properties of watermelon with the refreshing flavors of lime and mint. Watermelon is high in water content and rich in antioxidants, which promote hydration and overall well-being. Lime juice adds a zesty kick and alkalizing benefits, while fresh mint leaves provide a refreshing taste.

❖ Beetroot-Carrot Detox Elixir Ingredients:

- 1 small beetroot (rich in antioxidants and supports detoxification)

- 2 medium-sized carrots (packed with beta-carotene and vitamin A)

- 1 small apple (provides natural sweetness and fiber)

- 1-inch piece of ginger root (anti-inflammatory and aids digestion)

- 1 tablespoon lemon juice (cleansing and alkalizing)

- 1 cup filtered water

- Ice cubes (optional)

Instructions:

1. Wash and peel the beetroot, carrots, and apple.

2. Cut them into small pieces.

3. Peel the ginger root.

4. Add the beetroot, carrots, apple, ginger root, lemon juice, and filtered water to a blender.

5. Blend until smooth and well combined.

6. If desired, add ice cubes for a refreshing chill.

7. Pour into a glass and enjoy immediately.

Benefits: This detox elixir combines the cleansing properties of beetroot, carrots, apple, and ginger for a refreshing and detoxifying drink. Beetroot is rich in antioxidants and supports detoxification processes in the body. Carrots provide beta-carotene and vitamin A for overall well-being, while apple adds natural sweetness and fiber. Ginger root aids digestion and adds a spicy kick, while lemon juice provides cleansing and alkalizing benefits.

❖ **Mango-Coconut Antioxidant Delight**
   Ingredients:

- 1 ripe mango (high in antioxidants and vitamin C)

- 1/2 cup coconut milk (rich in healthy fats and creamy texture)

- 1 small ripe banana (provides creaminess and potassium)

- 1 tablespoon shredded coconut (optional for added flavor and texture)

- 1 tablespoon lime juice (refreshing and alkalizing)

- Ice cubes (optional)

Instructions:

1. Peel the mango and remove the pit.

2. Add the mango flesh, coconut milk, banana, shredded coconut (if using), lime juice, and ice cubes (if using) to a blender.

3. Blend until smooth and well combined.

4. Pour into a glass and serve immediately.

Benefits: This delightful smoothie combines the tropical flavors of mango and coconut for a refreshing and antioxidant-rich drink. Mango is high in antioxidants and vitamin C, which supports a healthy immune system. Coconut milk provides healthy fats and a creamy texture, while banana adds creaminess and potassium. Shredded coconut adds flavor and texture, and lime juice adds a zesty kick.

❖ Blueberry-Walnut Brain Booster Ingredients:

- 1 cup blueberries (rich in antioxidants and brain-boosting properties)

- 1/4 cup walnuts (high in omega-3 fatty acids and supports brain health)

- 1 small ripe banana (provides creaminess and potassium)

- 1 cup almond milk (or other plant-based milk)

- 1 tablespoon honey or maple syrup (optional for added sweetness)

- Ice cubes (optional)

Instructions:

1. Wash the blueberries thoroughly.

2. Add the blueberries, walnuts, banana, almond milk, and sweetener (if using) to a blender.

3. Blend until smooth and well combined.

4. If desired, add ice cubes for a refreshing chill.

5. Pour into a glass and enjoy immediately.

Benefits: This brain-boosting smoothie combines the antioxidant power of blueberries with the omega-3 fatty acids from walnuts. Blueberries are rich in antioxidants that protect the brain from oxidative stress and improve cognitive function. Walnuts contain omega-3 fatty acids, which support brain health and memory. The banana adds creaminess and potassium, while almond milk serves as a nutritious base. The optional sweetener enhances the taste.

❖ Kale-Pineapple Digestive Cleanse Ingredients:

- 2 cups kale leaves (packed with vitamins, minerals, and fiber)

- 1 cup pineapple chunks (contains bromelain for digestion)

- 1 small cucumber (hydrating and aids detoxification)

- 1 small piece of ginger root (anti-inflammatory and aids digestion)

- 1 tablespoon lemon juice (cleansing and alkalizing)

- 1 cup filtered water

- Ice cubes (optional)

Instructions:

1. Wash the kale leaves thoroughly.

2. Cut the pineapple into small chunks.

3. Peel and slice the cucumber.

4. Peel the ginger root.

5. Add the kale leaves, pineapple chunks, cucumber slices, ginger root, lemon juice, filtered water, and ice cubes (if using) to a blender.

6. Blend until smooth and well combined.

7. Pour into a glass and serve immediately.

Benefits: This digestive cleanse smoothie combines the nutrient-packed kale with the digestive benefits of pineapple, cucumber, ginger, and lemon. Kale is rich in vitamins, minerals, and fiber, promoting digestive health. Pineapple contains bromelain, an enzyme that aids digestion. Cucumber helps hydrate and detoxify the body, while ginger root reduces inflammation and aids digestion. Lemon juice provides cleansing and alkalizing benefits.

❖ **Turmeric-Ginger Immune Booster Ingredients:**

- 1 cup coconut water (hydrating and rich in electrolytes)

- 1 small ripe banana (provides creaminess and potassium)

- 1-inch piece of turmeric root (anti-inflammatory and immune-boosting)

- 1-inch piece of ginger root (anti-inflammatory and aids digestion)

- 1 tablespoon honey or maple syrup (optional for added sweetness)

- Ice cubes (optional)

Instructions:

1. Peel and slice the turmeric and ginger roots.

2. Add the coconut water, banana, turmeric root, ginger root, and sweetener (if using) to a blender.

3. Blend until smooth and well combined.

4. If desired, add ice cubes for a refreshing chill.

5. Pour into a glass and enjoy immediately.

Benefits: This immune-boosting smoothie combines the anti-inflammatory properties of turmeric and ginger with the hydrating benefits of coconut water. Turmeric contains curcumin, a compound known for its immune-boosting effects. Ginger root reduces inflammation and aids digestion. Banana adds creaminess and potassium, while coconut water replenishes electrolytes. The optional sweetener enhances the taste.

❖ Papaya-Mint Digestive Soother Ingredients:

- 1 cup ripe papaya chunks (rich in digestive enzymes)
- 1 small cucumber (hydrating and aids digestion)
- 1 tablespoon fresh mint leaves
- 1 tablespoon lime juice (refreshing and alkalizing)
- 1 cup filtered water
- Ice cubes (optional)

Instructions:

1. Cut the papaya into small chunks, removing the seeds.
2. Peel and slice the cucumber.
3. Add the papaya chunks, cucumber slices, fresh mint leaves, lime juice, filtered water, and ice cubes (if using) to a blender.
4. Blend until smooth and well combined.
5. Pour into a glass and serve immediately.

Benefits: This digestive soother smoothie combines the digestive enzymes of papaya with the hydrating properties of cucumber and refreshing flavors of mint and lime. Papaya contains papain, a digestive enzyme that aids in breaking down proteins and supports digestion. Cucumber helps hydrate and detoxify the body, while mint leaves add a fresh taste. Lime juice provides a zesty kick and alkalizing benefits.

❖ **Matcha-Green Tea Antioxidant Boost**
   Ingredients:

- 1 teaspoon matcha powder (packed with antioxidants)

- 1 cup brewed green tea (rich in antioxidants and boosts metabolism)

- 1 small ripe banana (provides creaminess and potassium)

- 1 tablespoon honey or maple syrup (optional for added sweetness)

- Ice cubes (optional)

Instructions:

1. In a cup, whisk the matcha powder with a small amount of hot water to form a paste.

2. Brew green tea according to package instructions and let it cool.

3. Add the matcha paste, brewed green tea, banana, and sweetener (if using) to a blender.

4. Blend until smooth and well combined.

5. If desired, add ice cubes for a refreshing chill.

6. Pour into a glass and enjoy immediately.

Benefits: This antioxidant-boosting smoothie combines the powerful antioxidants of matcha and green tea for a healthy and energizing drink. Matcha powder is rich in antioxidants called catechins, which help fight against free radicals in the body. Green tea is also packed with antioxidants and boosts metabolism. Banana adds creaminess and potassium, while the optional sweetener enhances the taste.

❖ **Tomato-Basil Cancer-Fighting Elixir**
   Ingredients:

- 2 ripe tomatoes (rich in lycopene, a powerful antioxidant)

- 1 small cucumber (hydrating and aids detoxification)

- 1 cup fresh basil leaves (packed with antioxidants and anti-inflammatory compounds)

- 1 tablespoon lemon juice (cleansing and alkalizing)

- 1 tablespoon extra-virgin olive oil (healthy fats)

- 1 cup filtered water

- Ice cubes (optional)

Instructions:

1. Wash the tomatoes and cucumber.

2. Cut the tomatoes into quarters and remove the core.

3. Peel and slice the cucumber.

4. Add the tomatoes, cucumber slices, fresh basil leaves, lemon juice, olive oil, filtered water, and ice cubes (if using) to a blender.

5. Blend until smooth and well combined.

6. Pour into a glass and serve immediately.

Benefits: This cancer-fighting elixir combines the antioxidant properties of tomatoes, cucumber, and basil. Tomatoes are rich in lycopene, a powerful antioxidant known for its potential to reduce the risk of certain cancers. Cucumber helps hydrate and detoxify the body, while basil leaves provide additional antioxidants and anti-inflammatory compounds. Lemon juice adds cleansing and alkalizing benefits, and olive oil contributes healthy fats.

❖ Avocado-Spinach Superfood Blend
Ingredients:

- 1 ripe avocado (packed with healthy fats and antioxidants)

- 2 cups fresh spinach leaves (rich in vitamins and minerals)

- 1 small ripe banana (provides creaminess and potassium)

- 1 tablespoon almond butter (or any nut butter of your choice)

- 1 tablespoon chia seeds (source of omega-3 fatty acids and fiber)

- 1 cup almond milk (or other plant-based milk)

- Ice cubes (optional)

Instructions:

1. Cut the avocado in half, remove the pit, and scoop out the flesh.

2. Wash the spinach leaves thoroughly.

3. Add the avocado flesh, spinach leaves, banana, almond butter, chia seeds, almond milk, and ice cubes (if using) to a blender.

4. Blend until smooth and well combined.

5. Pour into a glass and enjoy immediately.

Benefits: This superfood blend combines the nutritional power of avocado and spinach for a nutrient-dense smoothie. Avocado provides healthy fats and antioxidants, promoting heart health and overall well-being. Spinach is rich in vitamins and minerals, supporting a healthy immune system. Banana adds creaminess and potassium, while almond butter and chia seeds contribute additional healthy fats and fiber. The almond milk serves as a creamy and nutritious base.

❖ **Raspberry-Broccoli Antioxidant Blast
Ingredients:**

- 1 cup fresh or frozen raspberries (high in antioxidants and vitamin C)

- 1 cup broccoli florets (packed with antioxidants and fiber)

- 1 small ripe banana (provides creaminess and potassium)

- 1 tablespoon flaxseeds (source of omega-3 fatty acids and fiber)

- 1 cup coconut water (hydrating and rich in electrolytes)

- Ice cubes (optional)

Instructions:

1. Wash the raspberries and broccoli florets.

2. Cut the broccoli into smaller florets.

3. Add the raspberries, broccoli florets, banana, flaxseeds, coconut water, and ice cubes (if using) to a blender.

4. Blend until smooth and well combined.

5. Pour into a glass and serve immediately.

Benefits: This antioxidant blast smoothie combines the antioxidant power of raspberries and broccoli for a nutritious and flavorful drink. Raspberries are rich in antioxidants and vitamin C, which support a healthy immune system. Broccoli provides antioxidants and fiber, promoting overall health. Banana adds creaminess and potassium, while flaxseeds contribute omega-3 fatty acids and fiber. Coconut water helps hydrate and replenish electrolytes.

❖ Mango-Turmeric Energizing Blend Ingredients:

- 1 ripe mango (rich in vitamins and antioxidants)

- 1-inch piece of turmeric root (anti-inflammatory and immune-boosting)

- 1 small orange (source of vitamin C)

- 1 tablespoon hemp seeds (source of plant-based protein and omega-3 fatty acids)

- 1 cup coconut water (hydrating and rich in electrolytes)

- Ice cubes (optional)

Instructions:

1. Peel and dice the ripe mango.

2. Peel and slice the turmeric root.

3. Peel and segment the orange.

4. Add the diced mango, turmeric root, orange segments, hemp seeds, coconut water, and ice cubes (if using) to a blender.

5. Blend until smooth and well combined.

6. Pour into a glass and enjoy immediately.

Benefits: This energizing blend combines the tropical flavors of mango and the health benefits of turmeric. Mango is rich in vitamins, antioxidants, and dietary fiber, promoting overall health. Turmeric root provides anti-inflammatory and immune-boosting properties. Orange adds a burst of vitamin C, while hemp seeds contribute plant-based protein and omega-3 fatty acids. Coconut water helps hydrate and replenish electrolytes.

❖ Pomegranate-Berry Antioxidant Burst
   Ingredients:

- 1 cup pomegranate seeds (packed with antioxidants)

- 1 cup mixed berries (such as strawberries, blueberries, and raspberries)

- 1 small ripe banana (provides creaminess and potassium)

- 1 tablespoon honey or maple syrup (optional for added sweetness)

- 1 cup almond milk (or other plant-based milk)

- Ice cubes (optional)

Instructions:

1. Extract the pomegranate seeds from the pomegranate.

2. Wash the mixed berries.

3. Add the pomegranate seeds, mixed berries, banana, sweetener (if using), almond milk, and ice cubes (if using) to a blender.

4. Blend until smooth and well combined.

5. Pour into a glass and serve immediately.

Benefits: This antioxidant burst smoothie combines the vibrant flavors of pomegranate and mixed berries for a refreshing and antioxidant-rich drink. Pomegranate seeds are packed with antioxidants that help fight free radicals in the body. Mixed berries, including strawberries, blueberries, and raspberries, provide additional antioxidants and essential nutrients. Banana adds creaminess and potassium, while almond milk serves as a nutritious base. The optional sweetener enhances the taste.

❖ Blueberry-Spinach Brain Booster Ingredients:

- 1 cup fresh or frozen blueberries (packed with antioxidants and brain-boosting properties)

- 2 cups fresh spinach leaves (rich in vitamins and minerals)

- 1 small ripe banana (provides creaminess and potassium)

- 1 tablespoon almond butter (or any nut butter of your choice)

- 1 tablespoon honey or maple syrup (optional for added sweetness)

- 1 cup almond milk (or other plant-based milk)

- Ice cubes (optional)

Instructions:

1. Wash the blueberries and spinach leaves.

2. Add the blueberries, spinach leaves, banana, almond butter, sweetener (if using), almond milk, and ice cubes (if using) to a blender.

3. Blend until smooth and well combined.

4. Pour into a glass and serve immediately.

Benefits: This brain-boosting smoothie combines the antioxidant power of blueberries and the nutritional benefits of spinach. Blueberries are known for their high antioxidant content, which helps protect brain cells from oxidative stress and supports cognitive function. Spinach is rich in vitamins and minerals, promoting overall brain health. Banana adds creaminess and potassium, while almond butter provides healthy fats and additional nutrients. The optional sweetener enhances the taste.

❖ Beetroot-Carrot Blood Cleanser Ingredients:

- 1 small beetroot (rich in antioxidants and supports detoxification)

- 2 medium carrots (packed with vitamins and beta-carotene)

- 1 small apple (provides sweetness and additional antioxidants)

- 1 tablespoon fresh lemon juice (cleansing and alkalizing)

- 1 cup filtered water

- Ice cubes (optional)

Instructions:

1. Wash the beetroot, carrots, and apple.

2. Peel and chop the beetroot, carrots, and apple into smaller pieces.

3. Add the chopped beetroot, carrots, apple, lemon juice, filtered water, and ice cubes (if using) to a blender.

4. Blend until smooth and well combined.

5. Pour into a glass and enjoy immediately.

Benefits: This blood-cleansing smoothie combines the detoxifying properties of beetroot and the nutritional benefits of carrots and apple. Beetroot contains antioxidants that help cleanse the blood and support liver function. Carrots are rich in vitamins and beta-carotene, promoting overall health. Apple adds natural sweetness and additional antioxidants. Lemon juice provides a cleansing and alkalizing effect. The filtered water serves as a hydrating base.

❖ **Ginger-Turmeric Immune Booster Ingredients:**

- 1-inch piece of ginger root (anti-inflammatory and immune-boosting)

- 1-inch piece of turmeric root (anti-inflammatory and antioxidant-rich)

- 1 small orange (source of vitamin C)

- 1 small carrot (packed with vitamins and beta-carotene)

- 1 tablespoon fresh lemon juice (cleansing and alkalizing)

- 1 cup coconut water (hydrating and rich in electrolytes)

- Ice cubes (optional)

Instructions:

1. Peel and slice the ginger and turmeric roots.

2. Peel and chop the carrot.

3. Peel and segment the orange.

4. Add the sliced ginger, sliced turmeric, chopped carrot, orange segments, lemon juice, coconut water, and ice cubes (if using) to a blender.

5. Blend until smooth and well combined.

6. Pour into a glass and enjoy immediately.

Benefits: This immune-boosting smoothie combines the powerful properties of ginger and turmeric to support a healthy immune system. Ginger and turmeric roots are well-known for their anti-inflammatory and antioxidant benefits. Carrot provides vitamins and beta-carotene, while orange adds a dose of vitamin C. Lemon juice cleanses and alkalizes, and coconut water hydrates and replenishes electrolytes.

❖ Kale-Avocado Detox Blend Ingredients:

- 2 cups fresh kale leaves (rich in vitamins, minerals, and antioxidants)

- 1 ripe avocado (packed with healthy fats and antioxidants)

- 1 small cucumber (hydrating and aids detoxification)

- 1 tablespoon fresh lime juice (cleansing and alkalizing)

- 1 tablespoon chia seeds (source of omega-3 fatty acids and fiber)

- 1 cup coconut water (hydrating and rich in electrolytes)

- Ice cubes (optional)

Instructions:

1. Wash the kale leaves and cucumber.

2. Remove the tough stems from the kale leaves.

3. Peel and slice the cucumber.

4. Cut the avocado in half, remove the pit, and scoop out the flesh.

5. Add the kale leaves, avocado flesh, cucumber slices, lime juice, chia seeds, coconut water, and ice cubes (if using) to a blender.

6. Blend until smooth and well combined.

7. Pour into a glass and serve immediately.

Benefits: This detox blend combines the detoxifying properties of kale and cucumber with the nourishing benefits of avocado. Kale is packed with vitamins, minerals, and antioxidants that support overall health. Cucumber helps hydrate the body and aids in detoxification. Avocado provides healthy fats and antioxidants. Lime juice adds a cleansing and alkalizing effect. Chia seeds contribute omega-3 fatty acids and fiber. Coconut water serves as a hydrating base.

❖ **Pineapple-Green Tea Antioxidant Boost**
  Ingredients:

- 1 cup fresh pineapple chunks (rich in bromelain and antioxidants)

- 1 cup brewed green tea (packed with antioxidants)

- 1 small cucumber (hydrating and aids detoxification)

- 1 tablespoon fresh mint leaves (refreshing and aids digestion)

- 1 tablespoon honey or maple syrup (optional for added sweetness)

- Ice cubes (optional)

Instructions:

1. Peel and chop the pineapple into chunks.

2. Brew a cup of green tea and let it cool.

3. Wash and slice the cucumber.

4. Add the pineapple chunks, green tea, cucumber slices, fresh mint leaves, sweetener (if using), and ice cubes (if using) to a blender.

5. Blend until smooth and well combined.

6. Pour into a glass and serve immediately.

Benefits: This antioxidant boost smoothie combines the tropical flavors of pineapple with the health benefits of green tea. Pineapple contains bromelain, an enzyme that supports digestion and provides antioxidant properties. Green tea is rich in antioxidants, which help protect the body from oxidative stress. Cucumber adds hydration and aids in detoxification. Fresh mint leaves add a refreshing flavor, and the optional sweetener enhances the taste.

❖ Cherry-Walnut Recovery Blend Ingredients:

- 1 cup fresh or frozen cherries (packed with antioxidants)

- 1 small ripe banana (provides creaminess and potassium)

- 1 tablespoon walnuts (source of healthy fats and antioxidants)

- 1 tablespoon hemp seeds (source of plant-based protein and omega-3 fatty acids)

- 1 cup almond milk (or other plant-based milk)

- Ice cubes (optional)

Instructions:

1. Wash the cherries.

2. Remove the pits from the cherries.

3. Peel and slice the banana.

4. Add the cherries, banana slices, walnuts, hemp seeds, almond milk, and ice cubes (if using) to a blender.

5. Blend until smooth and well combined.

6. Pour into a glass and enjoy immediately.

Benefits: This recovery blend smoothie combines the antioxidant power of cherries with the nutritional benefits of walnuts. Cherries are rich in antioxidants that help fight inflammation and support recovery. Banana adds creaminess and potassium, while walnuts provide healthy fats and antioxidants. Hemp seeds contribute plant-based protein and omega-3 fatty acids. Almond milk serves as a creamy and nutritious base.

❖ Mango-Carrot Glow Booster Ingredients:

- 1 ripe mango (rich in vitamins and antioxidants)
- 2 medium carrots (packed with vitamins and beta-carotene)
- 1 small orange (source of vitamin C)
- 1 tablespoon fresh ginger (anti-inflammatory and immune-boosting)
- 1 tablespoon chia seeds (source of omega-3 fatty acids and fiber)
- 1 cup coconut water (hydrating and rich in electrolytes)
- Ice cubes (optional)

Instructions:

1. Peel and dice the ripe mango.

2. Wash and chop the carrots into smaller pieces.

3. Peel and segment the orange.

4. Peel and grate the fresh ginger.

5. Add the diced mango, chopped carrots, orange segments, grated ginger, chia seeds, coconut water, and ice cubes (if using) to a blender.

6. Blend until smooth and well combined.

7. Pour into a glass and serve immediately.

Benefits: This glow booster smoothie combines the tropical flavors of mango with the skin-nourishing benefits of carrots and orange. Mango is rich in vitamins, antioxidants, and dietary fiber, promoting overall skin health. Carrots provide a good dose of vitamins and beta-carotene, which helps maintain healthy skin. Orange adds a burst of vitamin C, while ginger adds anti-inflammatory and immune-boosting properties. Chia seeds contribute omega-3 fatty acids and fiber, while coconut water provides hydration and electrolytes.

= THE END =

We appreciate you selecting this book! We hope your expectations were fulfilled or surpassed.

Please think about posting a review on social media if you liked our book. We value your opinion because it enables us to make improvements to our goods and services for future clients.

We want to thank you once more for your support and send our best to you.

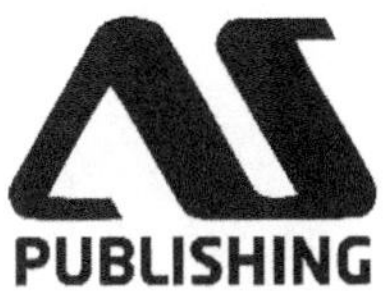

Follow Us to Stay Updated on New Releases

We offer our eBooks for free during the initial launch period. By following us, you will be among the first to know when a new eBook is released and have the opportunity to download it completely free of charge.

Don't miss out on our latest releases! Simply click on the link below, follow us, and stay up-to-date on all of our new eBooks.

amazon.com/author/as-publishing